Pegan Diet

Healthy And Delicious Recipes Perfectly Created To
Maximize The Paleo And Vegan Diets

*(Combining The Best Of The Paleo Diet And Vegan Diet For
Lifelong Health)*

Darrell Brandt

TABLE OF CONTENT

Introduction

Vegetables are inherently low in carbohydrates, but most of us consume too many. Obtaining enough protein is one of the greatest obstacles for those on vegetarian and vegan diets. This post is all about the Pegan diet, a method to obtain all the necessary nutrients while avoiding flesh.

Pegan means "Paleo" and "Vegetarian"; it is essentially a hybrid between two well-known low-carb diets aimed at achieving weight loss without sacrificing health benefits. This means that supporters may consume as much natural product as they desire, but should avoid carbohydrates such as pure sweetener and honey. Additionally, supporters may consume wine and other cocktails in moderation.

However, adherents are prohibited from consuming dairy products and processed foods. This is due to the fact that these foods are excessively high in carbohydrates and contain a great deal of unhealthy lipids, such as saturated fats. If all else is equal, adherents should consume as much conventional meat and vegetables as is reasonable, but no junk food.

The Pegan diet also differs from the Paleo and Vegetarian diets in that adherents may obtain their protein from any Along these lines source. In contrast to paleo dieters, who typically consume pork and poultry, Pegans may consume hamburger and other red meats.

The Pegan diet has many health benefits. Above all else, adherents are expected to experience weight loss benefits. This is due to the fact that the diet allows adherents to enjoy delicious, healthy lipids from grass-fed meats and omega-3 unsaturated fats from salmon. Paleo devotees cannot consume that!

However, it's not just about weight loss; it's also about enhancing general health. The rationale for this is that devotees are exhorted not to consume processed foods and dairy products, which frequently contain undesirable ingredients such as sugar and saturated fats.

In addition to consuming red meat, adherents can also consume other sources of protein, such as chicken and fish, which contributes to their superior health. It is impossible to obtain all of your protein from vegetables alone; they simply are not protein-rich enough.

Additionally, the Pegan diet is an excellent approach for managing a variety of diseases caused by consuming animal-based meats and animal lipids. These include coronary disease, joint pain, high cholesterol, and other diseases.

Obviously, the food sources you consume are also important. On a Pegan diet, adherents should consume an abundance of vegetables, as the majority of carbohydrates in a meat-based diet are typically derived from these foods. Additionally, it is essential to consume enough protein, vitamins, and minerals. This is the reason why it is essential to supplement this diet with a multivitamin.

There are additional benefits of adopting a Pegan lifestyle beyond weight loss and health enhancements. These can include a better night's sleep, enhanced mental clarity, and more.

To ensure that you receive all of the necessary nutrients and minerals, it is essential to consume a variety of foods. You crave an abundance of organic foods, vegetables, legumes, fish, and eggs. Additionally, it is recommended that you consume nutritious protein-rich foods such as chicken breast, eggs, and grass-fed beef.

There are certain foods that adherents of the Pegan diet should avoid. These include any processed or toxic foods, refined sugar, low-fat foods, and dairy products.

The Pegan regimen is simple to start and does not cost a lot of money. You will be required to purchase fresh produce and prepared proteins such as chicken and grass-fed beef, but you will have the option to prepare all of your meals at home.

THE PEGAN DIET

A

As its name suggests, the Pegan diet incorporates principles from both the paleo and vegan diets. How the world is it possible to combine two extremely restrictive regimens into one that is significantly simpler to follow?

Even though these two lifestyles are in opposition, the central concept emphasizes on reasonable and healthy food sources. The Pegan diet places a strong emphasis on foods derived from the earth and restricts processed food sources. In fact, Pegan diet adherents should concentrate on consuming 75% plant-based food varieties and 25% animal-based protein and high-quality lipids.

What Can I Consume on a Vegan Diet?

With the Pegan diet, it is optimal to adopt a plant-based mindset. Although meat consumption is permitted, it is not a central component of the diet. Meat is more of an appetizer or prelude to the star of the show, the main entree. Vegetables with a low glycemic index or those that are not monotonous are the primary components of the diet, along with an assortment of natural products. This regimen allows seeds such as almonds, pistachios, and walnuts, but peanuts should be avoided.

In addition to flax, chia, pumpkin, and other seeds, low-mercury fish such as sardines, herring, and anchovies are favored, as are salmon, anchovies, and mackerel. Consistently recollect natural, grass-fed beef, pork, and poultry are highlighted with regard to meat. Ensure that your protein sources are derived exclusively from grass-fed and antibiotic-free animals. Since eggs are a good source of essential nutrients and protein, they are permitted on this diet alongside heart-healthy oils like olive and avocado oil.

What foods am I to avoid?

Although the Pegan diet is generally not as restrictive as other weight loss plans, a few food types are excluded from this eating plan. Cow's milk-based dairy products, such as yogurt, milk, cheese, and butter, should be avoided under all circumstances. If you have a nut allergy, such as almond or coconut, you can consume small quantities of ewe or goat's milk. Similar to dairy, gluten is strongly discouraged; however, trace amounts of gluten-free whole cereals are permitted. Such dull vegetables as legumes are strictly prohibited.

If you have a craving for vegetables, lentils are optimal. Sugar should be used sparingly, and products with added sugar should never be consumed. The Pegan diet excludes vegetable oils such as canola, sunflower, maize, and soybean oil, as well as processed foods with artificial flavoring.

Should I Follow a Vegan Diet?

If dining like a cave dweller or restricting your diet to plants sounds challenging, you're not alone. It is! The Pegan diet permits the consumption of some meat, seafood, and eggs, but whole cereals, dairy products, and vegetables are restricted. Whether or not you should read the Pegan book depends solely on you. You obtained this book, so you have effectively taken a risk! You can start small by incorporating two or three Pegan meal plans into your weekly feast rotation and add more as you go.

As long as you consume more fruits, vegetables, plant-based protein legumes, unsweetened dairy products, and heart-healthy oils, you are on the correct path.

You will experience the advantages of a Pegan lifestyle if you make determined decisions to avoid indulging in pastries, doughnuts, and french fries.

Differences among Paleo, Pegan, and Vegan Diets

The entry point to the Pegan diet is the consolidation of Paleo and Vegan values. The Paleo diet requires adherents to consume only natural meats, poultry, seafood, organic products, vegetables, berries, and seeds. The Paleo Diet prohibits dairy products in addition to grains, vegetables, and processed foods.

For the vegetarian diet, adherents may consume fruits, vegetables, nuts, and seeds while avoiding all animal proteins and animal protein-containing foods such as milk and cheese.

When combining the Paleo and Vegan worlds, the resulting table of food options is particularly robust. On the Pegan diet, you can consume a broad variety of natural organic foods, vegetables, nuts, and seeds (similar to the Vegan diet), but also a limited amount of animal protein. While the Paleo diet eliminates all grains and vegetables, the Pegan diet allows for limited amounts daily.

Pegan Guidelines

Fruits, Veggies

On the Pegan diet, fresh vegetables and organic foods are always fashionable. You can consume a lot of raw or prepared vegetables, and fruits are great as well. However, you should limit fruits with a high sugar content, such as pineapple, because an inordinate quantity of sugar is unhealthy.

Seeds and Nuts

Nuts and seeds are rich in heart-healthy lipids and would have been an integral part of the Paleolithic diet. A daily serving of almonds and seeds will keep you satiated and provide the essential fatty acids for healthy skin, hair, and nails. However, keep in mind that it's simple to consume a large number of nuts and seeds, and despite the fact that it may seem like you've only consumed a small amount, nuts contain a large amount of oil in a small package. While consuming almonds, limit your intake.

Animal-Based Goods

Now that animal proteins are permitted on the Pegan diet, consider them as you would consider parsley when garnishing a dish; that is, the animal protein is not the main attraction on your plate, but rather somewhere between an embellishment and a condiment. Similarly, when selecting poultry, meats, and fish, ensure that they have been grain-fed or are untamed, respectively.

Eggs

The Pegan diet recommends consuming two eggs per day for protein and to ensure satiety so that you are not compelled to consume unhealthy foods.

Grains and Legumes

The Paleo diet excludes all grains and vegetables, but the advantage of the Pegan diet is that you can include small portions of both in your daily diet. Consistently consuming 12 cup of low-glycemic grains such as quinoa is recommended for satiety. Additionally, you can consume up to half a cup of vegetables daily for a protein boost.

The Pegan Distinction

Eating the Pegan way entails adopting healthy eating habits and consuming ideal, scrumptious food that is packed with all the nutrients you need. It is a well-balanced program that ensures adequate intake of all essential nutrients, from proteins to carbohydrates.

Eating the food sources that are most beneficial to your body also means that your body is better able to process them and convert them into the fuel it needs to remain healthy, happy, and energized.

YOUR GUT AND IMMUNE SYSTEM (CHAPTER 2)

You will be surprised to learn how much impact the digestive system has on the entire body. Unhesitatingly, we require additional pounds of food sources to be introduced directly into our gastrointestinal system multiple times per day. The digestive system is in charge.

Our capacity to convert the food we consume directly into fuel so that it can be absorbed and deliver various types of supplements. This will thus eliminate potentially hazardous substances from the body daily.

Consuming to Promote Digestive Health

Many of us have at one time or another considered discussing the microbiome. Currently, many aspects of our wellbeing and health, such as longevity and weight loss, can be degraded by our waste. As Hippocrates asserted, "all diseases begin in the digestive system," the statement is true. While the science behind understanding the microbiome is not at the expected level, experts in utilitarian medicine have routinely dealt with a wide range of persistent diseases, including chemical awkwardness, weight concerns, headaches, immune system disease, skin issues, malignant growth cells, cardiovascular infection, diabetes, disposition issues, sensitivities, and so forth. According to a specific study, it has been confirmed that a waste transfer can reduce the signs of chemical imbalance by 50%.

From this, it follows that the microbiome is likely the primary health regulator. In actuality, you will be astonished to learn that there are more than 100 trillion microbiomes in your stomach alone, which is nearly multiple times your DNA and multiple times the number of cells in your body. Similarly, our microbiome contains more than three million microbial genomes.

A third to half of the multitude of particles that remain in our blood originate from microbial metabolites, which are associated with virtually every interaction in our science, including brain science, the immune system, hormonal specialists, and qualities, among others. Our intestinal system microorganisms also provide us with essential nutrients such as biotin and vitamin K.

Nevertheless, our intestinal microbiome is not in the same condition as it once was.

Today, we are all too familiar with absurd medications, lifestyle choices, and food sources. We all consume a processed diet that is high in artificial additives, carbohydrates, and sugar, but to our dismay, roughly 70% of plants are sprayed with the microbiome-destroying herbicide glyphosate. Our diet is deficient in polyphenols and prebiotic filaments, both of which are required for the development of beneficial microorganisms. In addition, we take a great deal of stomach-damaging anti-inflammatory drugs, vitriolic blockers, and anti-microbial medications such as steroids, hormonal specialists, and Advil. From then on, we can include the impurities from the air, food, and water. Unfortunately, our body degenerates into a place filled with disease-causing agents and devoid of recovery agents. Inadequate food choices can lead to expansion, which is likely one of the primary causes of obesity and also persistent disease. Under a one-cell-thin stratum of the stomach lining, approximately 60 percent of the invulnerable framework exists in the intestinal tract. When subjected to severe treatment, this cell layer will unquestionably promote a damaged stomach, allowing microbial toxins, microorganisms, and dietary proteins to "leak" into the circulatory system. As the scientific community evolves, researchers and clinical experts are gaining a deeper understanding of the relationship between digestive dysbiosis and persistent illness. In fact, my personal experience left me terrified. Around twenty-five years ago, mercury damage to my gastrointestinal microbiome was so severe that I developed diarrhea, abdominal swelling, and irritable bowel syndrome. I have finally been able to eliminate mercury from my system and recover my intestines. Clearly, this was not the story's conclusion.

Prior to a few decades, the quality of focal points began to deteriorate. My initial incision was treated with the antibiotic clindamycin, which led to the development of a fatal infection in my intestines known as C. Diff, which kills approximately 30,000 individuals annually. My body was in agony around-the-clock, and there were also additional symptoms and manifestations such as vertigo, fever, loose intestines, bloody diarrhea, etc.

My gastrointestinal structure was in shambles! This continued for the subsequent five months, and I am currently unable to concentrate on my work. I also began taking high doses of the steroid prednisone in a misguided effort to get better, but it was ineffective.

Thankfully, I began utilizing the principles of utilitarian medicine as well as repairing my digestive system and recovering its function.

standard capability. The scientific investigation behind the microbiome has progressed to such a degree that I was able to construct a novel method to treat and prevent gastrointestinal issues.

My colitis disappeared within three weeks after I began to engage in it directly. I altered my dietary habits with the aid of various beneficial prescriptions. My method worked exceptionally well, and I am now able to treat every easily overlooked detail, including guiding meetings, irritable inside, and provoking gastrointestinal disease.

I started imagining my internal to be a solid and regulated nursery for the recuperation of my damaged digestive tract, which is the source of numerous persistent and incendiary diseases. It even helped me with excessive weight.

As soon as I imagined my digestive system as a nursery, I began utilizing three practices to cultivate a robust and balanced interior garden:

These ingredients are used to produce processed food sources that the American public is compensated for by the Food Stamp program. If a food company begins to fund a sustenance study, it is 50 times more likely that the study will demonstrate the food's benefit. Now that you have a thorough understanding of how the food industry operates, it is crucial that you choose an optimal diet. A pegan diet, as the name suggests, is a type of diet plan that adheres to the principles of both the paleo diet and the vegetarian diet. The Paleolithic era (more than 2.6 million years ago) was a time when meat, fish, vegetables, fruits, and seeds were readily available.

1. Consider over-the-counter drugs and foods as weeds. Therefore, the primary

step is to eliminate the following food types from your diet: Steroids

Antibiotic medications, unless absolutely essential

carbohydrates, particularly sugar alcohols and artificial carbohydrates like high-fructose corn syrup.

Dairy, gluten, and any other sensitive food varieties, such as legumes, cereals, and wheat, particularly if you have severe gastrointestinal dysbiosis.

Packaged or handled foods

Environmentally hazardous substances, such as maize, soy, and wheat; also avoid foods that have been sprayed with glyphosate Persistent pressure factors

Acid blockers

Anti-inflammatory drugs comparable to analgesics, such as naproxen (Aleve) and ibuprofen (Advil).

2. Add 'extraordinary annoyances' to your yard.

Once you have eradicated all of the harmful insects, it is time to introduce some beneficial insects to your garden, which include refined or aged food varieties such as:.

Unsweetened coconut yogurt Unpasteurized apple juice vinegar Regularly aged soy sauce Tofu (regularly aged) Tempeh (aged soy cake) Gluten-free tamari.

Miso.

Unsweetened kefir (preferably aged ewe or goat milk). Kimchi (aged vegetable or organic product) is fermented vegetables.

Sauerkraut that has developed naturally.

Next, you should take excellent care of your yard. You should consume foods that promote the development of substantial microorganisms in the intestines. Comprises of sources of fiber- and prebiotic-rich foods. Clinical specialists recommend introducing prebiotic foods progressively if you have a low number of digestive flora. If you consume a large number of prebiotic food varieties at once, the symptoms may become worse.

Some exceptional examples of prebiotic dietary varieties

consist of Algae. Bananas and plantains that are unripe.

Polyphenol-rich foods, such as climate-friendly tea,

Pomegranate as well as cranberry.

Leeks, garlic, and additionally shallots Jerusalem artichokes Jicama start. Asparagus Artichokes Dandelion Apples are climate-friendly. The following dietary sources are rich in fiber:

Strawberries.

Pumpkin Spinach.

Olive oil just as olives Lentils.

Nuts as seeds specifically produced figs. Kale

Celery Cucumber.

Cabbage and broccoli sprouts.

Beans Avocadoes Berries.

If you are struggling with a severe case of intestinal dysbiosis, I would recommend a fantastic beverage that will aid in the recovery of a wasteful digestive system. My colitis was cured in a short period of time. Due to thirty years of microbiome research, I concocted a drink that, in addition to healing my stomach, promoted the growth of healthy and balanced microorganisms such as Akkermansiamuciniphilus.

This particular microorganism maintains the physiological fluid and protects the layer to prevent a leaking digestive system. This microbe has been linked to cardiovascular disease, diabetes, obesity, immune system disorders, and even disease at low concentrations. If you do not have microorganisms in your framework, it is recommended that you avoid taking prebiotics. Flow research studies have demonstrated that Akkermansia thrives on the polyphenols found in green tea, pomegranate, and cranberry. In my case, polyphenols are the foundation for my inner yard. These micronutrients both nourish "incredible bugs" and rid my body of harmful microorganisms. Since I began experiencing this effect, I have been recommending the recipe for this shake to all of my family members and friends. When all else failed, this shake assisted me in treating my persistent condition. Additionally, it can be used to strengthen the intestine.

Here are the necessary ingredients for this smoothie.

A measurement of collagen powder.

A piece of your preferred high-potency probiotic (I used Xymogen's ProbioMax 350 DF).

A teaspoon of matcha climate-friendly tea powder, one tablespoon of concentrated cranberry juice, and one spoonful of concentrated pomegranate juice. One measure of acacia fiber.

An inside look at SBI Protect by NuMedicaImmunoG PRP. All you have to do is incorporate this assortment of ingredients with water to make a drink.

There is no doubt that practitioners of alternative medicine will be experts on digestive health. It makes no difference if you have a large amount of shock mercury in your system or are suffering from a parasite or infectious/bacterial overgrowth. A utilitarian medicine expert will examine your stomach wellbeing and health by analyzing your stool form, taking breath tests to look for an excess of negative irritants, and conducting food affectability tests in order to provide you with reasonable recuperation strategies and modified eating regimens. The vast majority of these specialists also offer instructive meetings, whether you choose to attend in-person or through online communication.

Consuming For The Immune System Of Your Body

The vast majority of us regularly forget that we have a resistant framework, recalling them only when something goes wrong, for example, when we get a flaw. Imagine the problems if our resistant framework only existed for the initial two or three weeks of the winter season. However, this framework is continuously at work to keep our bodies healthy, well-adjusted, and functional by fending off the unrelenting pressure of pathogenic organisms such as viruses and bacteria.

Yes, the body's immune system is adaptive, which means that there is always a possibility of something failing, ranging from minor irritations such as the common cold to immune system disorders such as Type-1 diabetes. Eventually, there will be a microorganism that will overcome your body's immune system and make you sickly.

Fortunately, there are a number of things you can do to ensure that your body's immune system continues to function normally for as long as possible; most of them do not involve medication. It has been determined that a paleo diet is sufficient to maintain the health of your body's immune system. This diet will reduce the stress that modern toxins have on your immune system, allowing it to focus on preventing infections such as the flu instead of wasting time with gluten in your bloodstream. When coupled with a healthy diet and sufficient rest, the body is constantly energized and prepared to deal with any type of antigen without the need for medication.

How exactly does the immune system function?

All organisms that cause infections, including microorganisms, infections, and parasites. Our body must eliminate antigens and other organisms from everything we imbibe, consume, contact, and ingest. If the person who contacted the handle before you has/had strep throat, streptococcus microorganisms have become a major problem for you.

Thankfully, our body is equipped with a high-tech device that aids in warding off microorganisms; without it, we would not have been healthy. The invulnerable framework is the first line of defense; an adaptable response is required for any potential threat. This includes the literal barriers to disease, such as the epidermis, as well as physiological fluid film layers for internal defense, such as the coating of the digestive system. This implies that the streptococcus organisms on the door handle must first enter the body before they can kill you. This severe inventory will be an ideal entry point for strep microorganisms due to the invulnerable framework.

Inside, the opposition framework will continue to protect you with the aid of nebulous protection tools such as expanding, which is a flexible form of safe criticism. Expanding will produce a real deterrent and release related synthetic compounds to entice phagocytes, a type of body-dwelling cells that will destroy intruders. While expanding may receive a great deal of negative press, particularly in the paleosphere, it is not entirely dangerous. Assuming it becomes a recurring problem, this is truly awful news.

Even if the microorganisms are able to breach this barrier, they will still be required to navigate the flexible safe framework. While the conventional immune system offers a one-size-fits-all approach, the adaptable immune system will provide antigen-specific responses. The intrinsic body invulnerability framework is largely determined by the qualities you inherit from your parents. In contrast, the individualized immune system will acquire immunity to a variety of infections that may have previously infected you. Although the response time is substantially lengthier, it is unquestionably more reliable.

White platelets, also known as lymphocytes, perform the most important role in a versatile immune system. They are formed in the bone marrow and divided into two major types: B cells (B lymphocytes) and T cells (T lymphocytes).

The B cells generate various types of antibodies. The next time you get strep throat, the b lymphocytes will immediately recall the streptococcus microorganisms and produce antibodies.

Antibodies are extraordinary, but you must eliminate the microorganisms to achieve excellence. There are two different types of T cells: the Helper T and the Awesome T. Paleo in addition to resistance.

Most types of diets contribute to immune system problems. A paleo diet will aid in the prevention and treatment of such conditions, including less prominent immune system issues such as psoriasis and skin inflammation. A paleo diet routine can also help strengthen the immune system by reducing the number of antigenic irritants such as influenza and colds.

This is a stricter version of the paleo diet, in which nightshade vegetables and eggs are eliminated. Additionally, you can reintroduce a few food sources after the conclusion of the introductory diet.

In addition to eradicating stomach noxious aggravations, a paleo diet includes food varieties that heal the stomach by restoring a healthy population of intestinal microorganisms. There are a few naturally fermented food varieties, for example, kefir, kimchi, and sauerkraut, that help repopulate beneficial microorganisms in the stomach, shield the stomach-related divider surface from a specific type of microorganisms, and diminish the harm of antibiotics. Experts have found that probiotics can aid individuals with Crohn's disease and hypersensitivities. A low-carb diet can also eradicate microbial overgrowth problems such as SIBO, which frequently causes digestive dysbiosis.

This does not imply that a zero-sugar diet is essential for immunity, particularly for those without digestive tract plant issues such as SIBO. A ketogenic diet will deprive the defenseless microorganisms, and there are also microorganisms that prefer ketones to sucrose. The immune system requires sugar to fend off foreign invaders; however, a persistent no-carb diet will unquestionably diminish the body's ability to respond to them.

Sugar is also required to maintain the membrane cell lining on the stomach lining, which is one of the primary actual antimicrobials that protect the intestinal tract from infection.

Certainly, this may be somewhat frustrating for you: Should you choose a diet in which ketosis helps treat an overabundance of microorganisms and increases the resistance of other microorganisms, or one in which the consumption of starch promotes the development of beneficial microorganisms and increases the resistance of other microorganisms? Fortunately, there are advantages to both types of diets, which can only be achieved by cycling sugar consumption.

For instance, you can practice intermittent fasting, which will provide you with the benefits of ketosis without requiring you to eliminate carbohydrates from your diet. In addition to providing you with the benefits of both a low-carb and a moderate-carb diet, consuming safe carbohydrates in moderation will supply your body with sugar when you are not fasting.

In addition, the nutrient content of your diet plays an important role in preserving a healthy immune system. Extreme deficiency in any one minor component can have observable effects on an invulnerable element, which is extremely common in developing nations.

Numerous individuals suffer from a variety of less severe deficiencies; this interaction between them can impair the normal presentation of the resistant trait.

Given the aforementioned, it is normal for you to seek out various types of beneficial Zinc or Vitamin C levels. Then again, consuming a healthy diet will ensure that your body's micronutrient levels are optimal.

In addition to diet, there are a number of non-dietary factors that can contribute to the development of high blood pressure. It will absolutely do wonders for your immune system!

A Summary Of The Pegan Diet

Due to the fact that the Pegan diet is quickly becoming an alternative diet for the majority of people who want to live a healthy lifestyle, several concerns and challenges have arisen regarding who should and should not use the Pegan diet. This is due to the fact that the Pegan diet as a lifestyle has generated a great deal of success, causing more people to want to jump on board. This includes individuals with a history of terminal ailments, underlying conditions, inherited diseases, and hypersensitivity.

Not everyone can be healthy by consuming vegetables, fruits, and lean proteins while avoiding dairy products. Aside from the most common problem of being unable to adhere to a diet, these substances simply impact individuals in very different ways. People with lactose intolerance may be pleased that the Pegan diet takes into account their allergy, whereas those with almond allergies may question what all the hubbub is about with the Pegan diet.

The query of who the Pegan regimen is best suitable for must therefore be answered. According to Hyman, the leading advocate of the Pegan diet, "the Pegan diet is not a passing fad that lasts a few days; it is a way of life." The context in which this query will be addressed can be deduced by analyzing Hyman's statement.

The Pegan diet is a sustainable, long-term approach to consuming and dieting that is beneficial for virtually everyone.

Before beginning the Pegan diet, however, individuals with a history of chronic ailments, including childhood maladies and medical conditions, must consult with their doctors and specialists. Associate Professor of Medical Oncology and Haematology at Oakland University- William Beaumont School of Medicine, Dr. Adil Akhtar, believes that the Pegan diet can be a healthy and balanced option for a large number of people, including those who are battling cancer or who want to reduce their risk of developing cancer.

According to Dr. Akhtar, the Pegan diet combines the positive aspects of the vegan and paleo diets to create a functional diet. Dr. Akhtar also recommends that individuals with even a hint of a specific health issue adopt a balanced diet abundant in vegetables and fruits and limit their consumption of processed foods and alcohol, which is the Pegan diet. People with an underlying ailment or a history of chronic illness can therefore begin the Pegan diet without risk. As a novice of the Pegan diet, the only thing you should do prior to changing your diet and if you have a specific illness is to obtain the advice of your physician, nutritionist, and dietician.

However, while the Pegan diet may appear to be the greatest development in the field of Nutrition in a very long time, it may not be an option for a few populations. Dr. Akhtar advises against beginning the Pegan diet for anyone struggling with an eating disorder, disordered eating patterns, or eating disorders that may be linked to a person's mental health. Although the Pegan diet has helped people lead healthier lives, it has not been scientifically proved to be the optimal diet; it is merely a fabricated eating plan.

On the other hand, encouraging individuals to adopt the Pegan diet by permitting the consumption of legumes and dairy products is also effective.

Even though the Pegan diet is not particularly restrictive, novices should not rush to find the ideal meal plan. Give it some time, and begin by consuming fruits and vegetables that you are already familiar with. Then, begin to increase the portion size of vegetables in your meals while decreasing your intake of carbohydrates, toxic lipids, and processed foods. The objective of the Pegan diet is to enhance the quality of your food and ensure that you consume dishes with an exceptionally high nutritional value.

As the Pegan diet gains more adherents, it faces greater opposition from those who wish to begin a diet or have already begun one. The exclusion of dairy products and cereals from the Pegan diet raises grave concerns. These concerns stem from the reality that while cereals and dairy products may not be entirely healthful, they do contain essential nutrients for good health. The issue then becomes, should the Pegan diet still be recommended? Or will a person on the Pegan diet lose out on certain nutrients? I will respond to this query in a variety of ways.

First, it is commonly believed that anyone on a diet is an adult, possibly over the age of 18. Everyone who desires to begin dieting is an adult with complete control over their bodies, decisions, and way of life. Milk, cheese, and butter contain vitamin A, folic acid, a substantial quantity of healthful lipids, and other nutrients. However, the continued consumption of these dairy products, particularly after the age of 40, poses a significant risk or challenge for many adults. This is because the energy and lipids obtained from dairy foods cannot be expended and exercised, or are rarely expended and exercised, due to this age group's apathy toward physical activity. Therefore, the absence of dairy foods in the Pegan diet is a method for preventing or reducing the accumulation of superfluous fat that is unlikely to be implemented.

The belief that much elderly individuals would be interested in trying the Pegan diet also helped to solidify this restriction. In recent years, however, it is not uncommon to see someone in their thirties on a diet. Thus, this concern persists.

As someone who has spent many years in nutrition as an advocate for proper dieting and a healthy lifestyle, I firmly believe that no one or object should limit you. You are not required to strictly adhere to the non-dairy and non-grain portion of the diet if you believe you still require a substantial amount of the nutrients in the diet. The purpose of avoiding dairy and gluten-containing grains is to prevent you from becoming nauseated after consuming them. The only consideration is that dairy, cereals, and legumes should be consumed in moderation, or they can be obtained from plants. For example, coconut produces coconut oil, coconut milk, and coconut butter. And these are ideal alternatives to dairy products. Because excessive consumption of dairy products may cause cancer and osteoporosis.

In essence, the Pegan diet excludes gluten-containing grains, legumes that may increase blood sugar levels, dairy products such as cow's milk, yogurt, and cheese, as well as sugar, refined oils and preservatives, and processed spices. However, a very small volume of these food groups may be consumed on occasion.

Many people have misconceptions about the Pegan diet, which leads them astray and prevents them from receiving the maximum benefits of the diet. The fact that the Pegan diet is a weight loss plan is one of them. That is utterly incorrect. The Pegan diet is a method for achieving and maintaining good health. It is not a quick fix for achieving "body goals" or losing weight.

Although there have been cases in which a person begins the Pegan diet and loses a significant amount of weight, including my own, it may not be a good idea to begin the Pegan diet if your goal is to lose weight. If you do not lose the desired amount of weight, you may become discouraged and even abandon the diet. And by doing so, you have probably deprived yourself of a very healthful lifestyle. It is true that the Paleo diet, which comprises a large portion of the Pegan diet, is well-known for promoting weight loss, but as a novice of the Pegan diet, you should not commence it with the intention of losing weight.

As previously stated, the Pegan diet is not a fad or a hobby; it is a lifelong commitment.

Despite the fact that the Pegan diet is rapidly gaining popularity and a growing number of people are adopting it, a large number of individuals are still unclear as to what the Pegan diet entails and what it actually achieves. To some, it is impossible to combine the Paleo diet with its time-honored practices and restrictions with the extremely restrictive Vegan diet. This group inquires about the feasibility of combining a diet that relies exclusively on legumes and cereals for protein with a diet that excludes beans and grains.

It is not only conceivable, but also yields incredibly beneficial results. Diets exist solely to provide individuals with the opportunity to practice and strive toward a healthful lifestyle. And the Pegan diet is not lacking in this regard. The Pegan diet is distinctive and adheres to its own set of rules. The primary focus is on vegetables and fruits, so you can always include a fruit or vegetable that was not specified in the meal plan or between the recipes for various dishes. However, consume more less acidic produce.

Meat consumption is also a part of the Pegan diet, albeit in small to moderate amounts, and meat and fish should be consumed with an abundance of vegetation. Nuts, seeds, and legumes are also integral components of the Pegan diet. While reading this, I want to ensure that you are already thinking about the meals you will incorporate into your plans and how you will initiate a fantastic Pegan diet. The Pegan diet is not ideal for those who want to try something new or different; it is a deliberate approach to living a healthy lifestyle.

The validity of the Pegan diet's main tenets has also been the subject of considerable debate. Due to its relative youth, the Pegan diet has not been scientifically validated in its genuine form. But a diet consisting of fruits, vegetables, a reduced quantity of locally produced livestock, nuts, seeds, and legumes is the most inclusive and comprehensive diet ever developed in the field of nutrition.

The benefits of a vegan diet are practically limitless. The Pegan diet ensures a very healthy existence by reducing the risk of cancer and other chronic diseases, promoting the respiratory system, and reducing inflammation. And at its current rate of effectiveness, the Pegan diet may still have many advantages.

Several concerns have also been expressed regarding the accessibility of the Pegan diet's goods. Some individuals may not have easy access to the majority of ingredients for some of the Pegan meal plan dishes. To comprehend this concern regarding lack of accessibility, it is essential to recognize that the proliferation of processed and packaged foods may make the majority of the Pegan diet's recommended food groups scarce. Even in adjacent shopping malls and supermarkets, fruits and vegetables on the shelves are rarely freshly produced. Additionally, flesh and fish were grown in one day and sold the next. Under the guise of fertilizers, many fruits and vegetables are produced and grown with a variety of chemicals. This could be a significant strain on the Pegan diet because, despite consuming healthily, you are uncertain as to whether you are actually healthy.

I will explain how I was able to overcome this obstacle on my own. Beginning the Pegan diet was relatively simple for me because I have always been a proponent of healthy eating, albeit with occasional lapses. So, when I began the Pegan diet, I discovered that the majority of the fruits, vegetables, legumes, gluten-free cereals, and other foods I had been purchasing and incorporating into my diet were actually not part of the diet. The Pegan diet prohibits the consumption of meat and other protein sources in their leanest forms, which I could not obtain at the mall. I began growing tomatoes, okra, green beans, and other green vegetables in a small garden on my front veranda.

If I were to prepare a salad for lunch, I had most of the necessary ingredients on hand. As soon as I realized this was effective, I expanded my "farm" to the rear of my home and began cultivating numerous other vegetables. I soon began cultivating berries in the backyard of my home! I would work all morning and then return home to prepare a fast meal before retiring to bed. I did not have to fret about the refrigerator and larder being supplied. I had practically everything I required nearby. My family pondered if I had developed a "obsession" with flora. However, this was not the situation. I was cultivating my own sustenance, and nothing could have been better. I took complete responsibility for what I ingested, and I never took it casually.

The Pegan diet, which adopts this aspect of the Paleo diet, stipulates that a greater proportion of the meat ingested must be pasture-fed and locally produced. Since I am not an animal lover and don't even own a companion, the notion of raising animals for food was out of the question. There may be several methods to accomplish this, but I began liaising with wholesalers and distributors of meat in my county and obtaining their suppliers' contact information in order to reach those who raised their animals locally. Obviously, I had to compensate them amply. I also reduced my protein intake when I was uncertain of their origins.

I also befriended local farmers who raised animals and became a regular at the abattoir, reaching out to those I trusted for freshly raised, nutritious meat. There are undoubtedly other methods to ensure you consume healthy meals, but this is how I overcame these obstacles.

The Significance Of Coupling Exercise And The Pegan Diet

In this section of the book, we will attempt to explain how sport can be of great assistance in achieving fundamental and advanced dietary objectives. Even more so in a Pegan diet. As with any regimen, exercise is a necessary, if not essential component. This is due to the fact that a caloric deficit is necessary for weight loss in order for the diet to function. Adding the calorie reduction from exercise to the calorie reduction from diet will increase the likelihood of observing this result. In addition, if we consider the application of sport to the Pegan diet in our particular case, we will have an essential contribution not only to weight loss but also to one of the greatest advantages of this diet. As previously stated, one of the primary advantages and characteristics of the Pegan diet is that it seeks to realign the diet in order to reset the metabolism. With the inclusion of sport, this process can be accelerated and completed more quickly.

Caution is advised, however, as it is not required that you are a super-athlete, particularly if you are in a regimen as restrictive as the Pegan diet. For this reason, we have decided to divide the Pegan diet, as a regimen for the fundamental sport, into a distinct paragraph from the specific tactics and enhancements for competitive athletes.

Returning to the discussion of the Pegan diet and exercise, we can relate to what has been stated previously and assert that this protocol must be accompanied by fundamental exercise. This means that when we discuss beginner sports to complement the Pegan diet, we are explicitly referring to novice sports. This regimen does not require you to be a professional marathon runner or cross-fitter, as it implies you require more macronutrients, such as carbohydrates.

Despite this, the sport we are discussing is the one that is typically played at home or in the park. Therefore, it is a completely free-body sport that will be useful for weight loss. A sport that requires excessive physical exertion, such as running or bodybuilding, is quite hazardous.

Regarding the latter, we have just mentioned that the training that should accompany this diet is free body training, or training without weights. However, lightweights are permitted but must be kept to a minimum.

In any event, integrating the proper physical activity with the Pegan diet is required for optimal results. We are not here to enumerate all the advantages of general physical activity, but we will list those that are compatible with the Pegan diet:

• Firstly, as we've already stated, the Pegan diet and exercise will create a specific caloric deficit for speedier weight loss.

• It will help you speed up your metabolism: we stated that the goal of this diet is to educate people about proper nutrition and thus reset a sluggish metabolism. Incorporating physical activity into your routine will accelerate your metabolism and produce long-lasting results.

• Combining sport with the Pegan diet will increase the health benefits: when discussing cardiovascular disorders or diabetes, we mentioned the role of the Pegan diet in containing and preventing the problem. Adding physical activity will have an even greater impact on blood insulin and glycemia levels, as well as the functioning of blood pressure.

After elaborating on the significance of sport in the Pegan diet, we'd like to provide you with some practical application advice, first for amateur athletes and then for professionals.

Advice for those who are novices in sports

We have stated that bodyweight training can be performed both at home and outside. Physical activity should not be overdone, as this is always a restrictive regime. This would only result in the danger of physical collapse.

Regardless, the following are some helpful guidelines for practicing sports while on a Pegan diet:

• Initially, always favor low-impact cardio exercises. This means that the ideal sport to practice while dieting remains activities that do not require inordinate exertion of the heart or lungs. In practice, these are all cardiovascular exercises with minimum impact, such as walking (slowly or quickly), stationary cycling, and cycling on flat terrain. All of these activities have a moderate calorie expenditure, so they will aid you in your diet without completely depleting your body's energy reserves for the day.

• Do not overdo it: you do not need to perform the activities every day. Two or three cardio sessions per week are sufficient. Obviously, we do not intend to discourage you from walking every day. In addition to its contribution to the diet, walking is beneficial for both the body and the mind.

• Do not even exceed the training time: an hour or an hour and a half is sufficient. As you are on a restrictive diet, doing more would be dangerous.

• If you decide to use weights regardless, avoid using an excessive burden. Lightweights with the appropriate reps are acceptable.

• Never neglect to perform muscle relaxation exercises: stretching is essential for relaxing and calming muscles.

• In relation to the preceding, yoga would be an ideal type of activity for a Pegan diet, as it does not require excessive exertion and will improve your mental and physical health.

These are the finest recommendations for the fundamental sport associated with the Pegan diet, which we have outlined above. Always refrain from overdoing it and consult a physician for specific instructions.

Tips for those who are competitive in athletics.

In the preceding paragraph, we provided you with the finest advice on noncompetitive sports and the Pegan diet.

Now we will discuss those who participate in competitive sports. We have decided to separate these two sections, as their levels of difficulty are vastly distinct. A first level of difficulty relates to the fact that an amateur who practices sport at a fundamental level will not exert the same effort or train with the same frequency as professionals.

If you are on the Pegan regime, we previously advised you not to overuse the frequency and hours of exercise. This is because you may not have sufficient vitality to sustain a greater or longer-lasting effort.

Consider the situation in greater detail if you must compete in a marathon or a professional sporting event that requires specific preparation and an optimal level of energy in the body.

In fact, a second level of difficulty is posed by the increased energy requirements of professional sport. Staying under the Pegan regime in its restrictive guise and engaging in heavier and more continuous sports remains an impossibility.

Nonetheless, we believe it is essential to develop some reasoning skills. As stated previously, sport and diet are two virtually unbreakable unions. If sport aids in dieting for the purpose of losing weight and altering the metabolism, then the correct diet aids in dieting for the purpose of having the best possible physical condition and enhancing one's professional performance.

What differs is the objective: in professional sport, it is assumed that weight loss is unnecessary, so the diet to be followed will only aid in achieving optimal physical fitness. Maximum physical condition does not correspond with actual weight loss.

However, what should you do if you wish to follow a wholesome diet to enhance your athletic performance?

First, the opinion of a medical nutritionist: if you are a professional athlete, consult your physician to determine if the diet is tailored to your requirements, if it is sustainable, and if it will actually help you achieve your goal.

In spite of this, you could never adhere to this diet in its most restrictive form. As stated previously, a person who engages in a great deal of sport requires a great deal of vitality. Known sources of energy include primarily carbohydrates. In this situation, a low-carb diet is not the best option. Nevertheless, with a few additional tips and techniques, the Pegan diet can be adapted for athletes who compete at a high level-

Therefore, to adhere to this regimen, you will need to take the following precautions:

• Initially, it will be necessary to increase the amount of carbohydrates consumed. In addition to proteins and vegetables, you will need to consume an equal quantity of carbohydrates. Always opt for whole cereals, legumes, and foods whose origins you are familiar with (avoid packaged munchies, industrial treats, and refined flours).

• Increase portion sizes: there is discussion of increasing portion sizes in general, especially if you engage in a strenuous sport and require a great deal of proteins and micronutrients. Therefore, you must not only include carbohydrates in your Pegan diet, but also enhance the amounts of meat/fish/eggs and vegetables.

• Do not overlook fruit: always of biological origin, fruit is an essential source of immediate energy for athletes. Additionally, it is abundant in essential vitamins and nutrients.

These precautions will be useful if you wish to adhere to a healthy diet and, at the same time, maintain ideal physical and athletic heath. This chapter on the relationship between the Pegan diet and sport concludes now. In the following chapter, we will demonstrate how this diet functions in practice, including which foods are permitted and which are strictly forbidden.

6. Say No to Vegetable Oils

Vegetable oils are detrimental to your health and the environment, a fact that is not widely known. Vegetable oils are oils extracted from various plants.

Nut, safflower, sunflower, corn, soybean, and rapeseed (canola oil) seed varieties. Unlike olive oil and coconut oil, which are extracted by pressing, these vegetable oils are extracted in an unnatural manner.

In addition to the persistent misconceptions about cholesterol and saturated fats, these oils are frequently promoted as healthful due to the omega-3 unsaturated fats and monounsaturated fats they contain. In the future, these fraudulent health claims will be a frequent focus. However, this does not explain the image as a whole.

The human body contains 97% polyunsaturated fatty acids (PUFAs), which are abundant in vegetable oils. saturated and monounsaturated lipids make up the remaining 3%. The fat is required for hormone production and cell maintenance. In contrast, PUFAs are extremely unstable and oxidize swiftly. This can subsequently lead to cell mutation and inflammation. The oxidation has also been linked to other cardiovascular diseases.

Omega-3 fatty acids are widely acknowledged to be exceedingly beneficial. Nevertheless, the ratio of omega-3 to omega-6 fatty acids is crucial for optimal health.

Many omega-6 fatty acids are present in vegetable oils. These acids undergo accelerated oxidation. However, it has been shown that omega-3 fatty acids protect against cancer and reduce inflammation. Unbalanced levels of both types of acids have been linked to several types of cancer and other health problems.

In addition to omega-6 fatty acids and polyunsaturated lipids, these vegetable oils contain chemicals, pesticides, and processing additives. Some also contain the natural antioxidants BHT and BHA, which prevent food from spoiling quickly. However, according to research, they also produce cancer-causing compounds in the body. Moreover, vegetable oil is linked to kidney and liver damage, behavioral issues, infertility, and immune system issues.

7. Abstain from sugar and eat fruits Moderately

From peanut butter to marinara sauce, nearly all products contain added sugar. The majority of individuals consume processed foods for snacks and dinner. These products contain added sugar, which significantly contributes to their calorie content.

According to dietary guidelines, you should consume no more than 10% of your daily calories from added sugar. It has been determined that excessive sugar consumption is the leading cause of obesity and can also contribute to a variety of chronic diseases, such as Type 2 diabetes.

The prevalence of obesity is at an all-time high, and sugar-sweetened beverages are a significant contributor. Fructose is a basic sugar found in sugar-sweetened beverages such as sweet tea, juice, and soda. When fructose is consumed, appetite increases. Additionally, fructose increases resistance to leptin, a hormone that regulates appetite and signals the body to cease consuming.

In brief, sugary beverages do not satisfy appetite, and you end up consuming excessive calories from liquids, leading to weight gain. According to research, those who consume sweetened beverages are heavier than those who do not.

A diet elevated in fructose can also increase the risk of developing cardiovascular disease. High-sugar diets have been linked to inflammation, obesity, and elevated blood pressure, all of which are risk factors for a variety of cardiac conditions.

Increased sugar intake has also been associated with acne. Foods with a high glycemic index, such as processed sweetened delights, raise blood sugar levels more rapidly than foods with a low GMI. These foods will cause insulin and blood sugar levels to rise, resulting in increased inflammation, sebum production, and androgen secretion, all of which contribute to acne. In addition, population studies have revealed that rural areas of the globe that ingest unprocessed foods have virtually no acne, compared to high-income areas and cities.

8. Avoid Gluten Grains

As stated previously, gluten is a naturally occurring protein present in cereals such as rye, barley, and wheat. This substance has a flexible aspect and is responsible for holding the meals together. Triticale, einkorn, Khorasan wheat, graham, farro, farina, semolina, emmer, durum, spelt, and wheat berries are additional grains that contain gluten. Although oats are innately gluten-free, cross-contamination occurs during processing with the cereals enumerated previously. Additionally, modified food starch and soy sauce are less apparent sources of gluten.

The downside of gluten is that it can induce adverse effects in some individuals. When the immune system recognizes gluten as a pathogen, it will launch an attack against it. If you are gluten-sensitive and accidentally consume gluten, you will experience inflammation. Mild side effects include diarrhea, alternating constipation, bloating, and fatigue, while severe side effects include intestinal injury, malnutrition, and unintended weight loss.

It has been estimated that one in 113 Americans suffers from celiac disease, and it has been determined that those with celiac disease have an increased risk of anemia and osteoporosis. This results in additional health issues, including nerve disorders, infertility, and even cancer.

The positive news is that the injury can be reversed by removing gluten from one's diet. A gluten-free diet is frequently the solution for celiac disease.

However, adhering to a gluten-free diet is not simple; you may need the assistance of a registered dietitian to determine which foods contain gluten and to find gluten-free substitutes for other essential nutrients.

In brief, a gluten-free diet is a diet that prohibits the consumption of gluten-containing foods. However, the majority of gluten-containing whole grains also contain iron, magnesium, and vitamins. Therefore, it is essential that you replenish these nutrients. For example, you can consider poultry, eggs, fish, legumes, and whole fruits and vegetables as inherently gluten-free foods.

9. Include Nutritious Fats

The majority of individuals are unable to comprehend why monounsaturated and polyunsaturated fats are beneficial to the body and why trans fats are harmful. In fact, we have been attempting to eliminate lipids from your diets whenever possible by recommending low-fat meals. However, this transformation does not enhance our health because beneficial lipids are reduced alongside unhealthy fats.

While some lipids are detrimental to the human body, others are essential. Fats are one of the most essential energy sources for the human organism. It will aid in mineral and vitamin absorption. Additionally, fats contribute to the formation of sheaths surrounding nerves and cell membranes. Additionally, fats are beneficial for inflammation, muscle movement, and blood coagulation. Consequently, certain lipids are beneficial to the organism in the long term.

All lipids, whether healthy or unhealthy, share a similar chemical structure. It is composed of a chain of carbon atoms and hydrogen atoms. The only distinction between these lipids is the number, size, and configuration of the hydrogen and carbon atoms, respectively.

Before discussing the excellent and healthy fats, let's examine the unhealthy fats. Trans fat is the most dangerous form of fat. This fat is produced when hydrogenation is used to transform healthful oils into solids to prevent rancidity. This form of fat has no health benefits and is also unsafe for consumption. In fact, trans fat has been prohibited in countries such as the United States.

In contrast, polyunsaturated and monounsaturated lipids are healthy fats found primarily in fish, seeds, almonds, and vegetables. At ambient temperature, this form of lipid remains liquid.

When you submerge your bread into olive oil, you consume monounsaturated fat. This fat contains a solitary carbon-to-carbon double bond, resulting in two fewer hydrogen atoms. Monounsaturated lipids remain liquid at ambient temperature for this reason. Sunflower oils, almonds, avocados, peanut oil, and olive oil are excellent sources of monounsaturated fats.

Consume Clean Meat, Poultry, and Whole Eggs

As previously stated, meat and poultry are excellent sources of protein for a Pegan diet. In addition, they contain many essential nutrients, such as essential fatty acids, vitamins, zinc, iron, and iodine. As a result, it is always advisable to include poultry, meat, and eggs in a Pegan diet. To avoid consuming saturated fat and sodium, however, it is recommended that you adhere to lean and unprocessed cuts.

Clean eating is an amorphous concept, signifying that there are no caloric or dietary restrictions. Avoiding packaged and processed foods that are high in artificial ingredients, sodium, and sugar appears to be the common denominator of clean eating when it comes to whole eggs, meat, and poultry. Thus, you choose whole or natural animal-based goods over processed ones.

Eggs, poultry, and meat should be purchased fresh, unseasoned, and free of artificial ingredients. These foods are nutritionally dense, high in protein, and minimal in fat by design.

After ensuring that you have purchased clean meat, cooking will eliminate all bacteria and other microorganisms. In addition to being nutritious, it will safeguard you and your family against food contamination.

Preparing To Go Pegan

Today, it is common for individuals to begin a Pegan diet; it is the newest diet trend. Can you consume meat? Yes, but you should not exaggerate.

What about manufactured substances? You can only consume a few. This diet consists primarily of whole foods, so you will consume fresh vegetables and fruits.

The Pegan diet is a combination of the vegan and paleo diets based on the theory that whole foods promote optimal health by reducing inflammation and balancing blood sugar.

Combining vegan and paleo diets may appear contradictory or strange at first sight. However, rest assured that this is not the case. You should view it as a compromise that combines the finest aspects of both regimens.

Meal planning is fundamentally straightforward. As stated previously, Pegan diet recipes include modest quantities of high-quality animal-based proteins, an abundance of healthful lipids, and fruits and vegetables. In addition, you must avoid legumes (peanuts, lentils, peas, and beans), cereals, and dairy products.

Vegan and paleo diets both adhere to the following program tenets:

Fats from olive oil, grains, almonds, avocados, and omega-3 fatty acids are of superior quality.

Consider organic, hormone- and antibiotic-free, and non-GMO foods as pesticide-free.

Absolutely no chemicals: No MSG, artificial colors, flavors, or additives.

Look for vegetables and fruits with intense and vibrant hues; the greater the variety, the better.

Low in refined carbohydrates, flour, and sugar

If you choose to follow the Pegan regimen, you will:

Consume saccharine products sparingly; you can enjoy them on occasion.

Avoid legumes, cereals, and dairy

Consume an abundance of seeds and almonds because their high protein content reduces the risk of diabetes and cardiovascular disease.

Vegetables should comprise approximately 75% of your daily diet.

Consume the proper lipids, such as omega-3, seeds, olive oil, almonds, and avocados; avoid soy and vegetable oils.

Consume foods with a low glycemic burden; instead, seek out more lipids and proteins in foods such as sardines, olive oil, seeds, and almonds.

Controversy

Since 2014, Pegan recipes and diet have risen dramatically in popularity. In 2021, Pinterest searches for 'consuming Pegan' increased by 337%. However, this regimen has also generated some controversy.

For instance, experts have suggested that the general parameters of this diet are merely the combination of two opposing diet philosophies. In reality, they believe that the majority of Pegan diet restrictions are time-consuming, expensive, and unnecessary.

According to these nutritional and dietary authorities, limiting legumes could be problematic, for instance. According to studies, legumes are low in cholesterol, high in fiber, and a rich source of protein, making them an essential component of the widely popular Mediterranean diet. In addition, legumes have been associated with numerous health benefits, including the prevention of cardiovascular disease, cancer, etc.

Optimistic Reports

While there have been some debates about the Pegan diet, there have also been numerous positive responses. The majority of experts concur with Dr. Hyman that animal-based products should be ingested as condiments and not as the primary course. Additionally, scientists adore the notion of increasing vegetable, fruit, and seafood consumption.

Others have concurred that there are numerous aspects of a Pegan diet, such as the emphasis on omega-3 fatty acids, fruits, and vegetables, and adequate protein. The conclusion is that a Pegan diet may be beneficial to your health. Nevertheless, there are certain restrictions that you must observe. If you can do so, the Pegan diet will begin to have a beneficial effect on your body.

The Pegan Grocery List

 Now that you know what to expect, here are a few items that should be at the top of your purchasing list:

Your diet should include vegetables with a low glycemic index or carbohydrate content, such as tomatoes, peas, carrots, broccoli, mushrooms, leeks, eggplant, peppers, cauliflower, Brussel sprouts, greens (turnip, mustard, collard, etc.), bamboo stalks, etc.

Look for fruits with a low starch or glycemic index, such as pineapple, mangoes, pears, citrus fruits, dark berries, cherries, apples, oranges, watermelons, etc. Purchase fruits with a high hydration content.

Animal Protein: As long as the flesh is grass-fed and sourced in a sustainable manner, you can consume animal proteins such as whole eggs, poultry, cattle, pork, venison, etc. Additionally, you can consume seafood such as shrimp and halibut.

Healthy Fats: For a Pegan diet, you must consume minimally processed fats from specific sources, such as nuts (except peanuts), seeds (except processed seed oils), unrefined coconut oil, olives, avocados (ensure the avocado and olive oil are cold-pressed), and omega-3 fatty acids (ensure the fish has a low mercury content).

Since you cannot consume dairy products, you are unable to consume conventional butter. There are numerous alternatives to butter, such as vegan butter and pureed avocado. In contrast, some varieties of oils include sesame oil, olive oil, and others. Avoid vegetable oils.

Dairy Replacement: For a Pegan diet, hemp, almond, soy, cashew, hazelnut, and oat are excellent dairy alternatives.

You can include natural carbohydrates such as vanilla, dates, honey, coconut sugar, and maple syrup in your diet.

Except for peanuts, most nuts, such as almonds and hazelnuts, can be ingested. Regarding seeds, chia, pumpkin, and flax seeds provide a nutritious boost.

While legumes are typically discouraged on the Pegan diet, gluten-free, whole legumes are still permitted in limited quantities. The daily allowance should not exceed 75 grams. Pinto legumes, black beans, chickpeas, and lentils are some examples.

Miscellaneous: You may include a variety of miscellaneous ingredients as long as they are natural and low on the glycemic index.

It is advised that you limit your consumption of starchy foods. Even if you consume starches, make sure they come from wholesome sources.

For baked goods, ensure that the ingredients do not contain refined sugar and are gluten-free. Additionally, you can include black rice, quinoa, oats, black beans, and chickpeas.

Supplements: In the case of a Pegan diet, you may take Vitamin D3 and omega-3 fatty acids as supplements. Also available is Vitamin B12.

Pegan Diet And Exercise

This diet involves not only consuming the correct combination of plant and animal foods, but also practicing in the proper manner. If you want to be healthy (and maintain a healthy weight), you must engage in cardiovascular and hebdomadal strength training practices four or five times per week, in addition to adhering to the Pegan diet plan requirements. The goal is to increase caloric expenditure by 300–500 calories per week by practicing for 30–60 minutes per day, five days per week.

Pegan Diet and Weight Loss Overview

Those adhering to the Pegan diet guidelines will typically experience rapid weight loss, with noticeable results typically visible within 2–3 weeks of following the diet plan. This feeding pattern has likely become one of the most recognizable in recent years. The focus is on reducing a person's weight while permitting them to consume energizing and nutritious meals and snacks.

Is the Pegan Diet a Good Option for You?

This diet comes after other diets with potential clinical benefits, most notably the paleo and vegetarian beloved diets, which count caloric. The Paleo diet emphasizes whole, natural dietary sources and animal products. On the other hand, you will consume substantially less meat (and presumably more natural items) on a Pegan diet than on a Paleo diet.

With its profusion of plant-based food options, this diet is closely related to veganism, which is also a lifestyle founded on specific natural principles and health concerns. The agnostic view of meat and the restriction of the majority of cereals and vegetables is regarded as superior. Depending on your tendencies, one may be easier for you to follow than the other.

This eating regimen additionally bears resemblances to the "wonderful eating" design, which regularly incorporates choosing whatever a few normal food assortments are permitted to be, regularly without pesticides or genetic modification. Additionally, the recorded Whole30 diet may be a 30-day start that appears almost identical to a Pegan diet, excluding dairy, cereals, and vegetables, according to various viewpoints. However, this diet is not merely similarly restrictive, as the Whole30 is intended to be followed until the end of the day.

A Pegan diet, which excludes cereals, legumes, and dairy products, must be balanced when compared to government guidelines for a healthy diet standard, because it is unbalanced. The USDA's 2020–2025 Dietary Guidelines for Americans recommend consuming a variety of nutrient-dense foods, such as fruits, vegetables, whole cereals, lean protein sources, low-fat dairy products, and healthy lipids, for a healthy diet.

Since a Pegan diet does not dictate how much you will consume on any given day, it does not conflict with the USDA's guidelines for daily calories, large scope, and micronutrients. You must choose to manage these issues with cautious planning while adhering to the diet's list of permitted food types.

Understanding your daily calorie requirements can help you maintain focus on your objectives if you're trying to get healthier. If you're interested in calorie monitoring, this analyst can offer you a measurement.

How Do The Operating Principals Operate?

The primary focus of the alkaline diet is alkaline-rich foods. Diet alone cannot readily alter the pH level of the blood. Geographic location has an effect on the pH of the body. The stomach is, among other things, significantly more acidic. I will then elucidate what I mean.

The pH scale ranges from 0 to 14, with 0 being the most basic and 14 being the most acidic.

The body's pH levels should remain constant.

When discussing the alkaline diet, it is necessary to understand pH.

pH is an analytical unit used to measure the acidity or alkalinity of a solution.

Between 0 and 14 is the pH scale's range:

Neutral: 0.0-6.7.0; alkaline or basic: 7.1-14.0.

Checking one's urine's pH (greater than 7) is a common recommendation made by proponents of this diet (below 7).

However, it is essential to remember that the pH of your body varies significantly. Body acidity and alkalinity are not defined.

The stomach's hydrochloric acid gives it a pH of 2-3.5, making it extremely acidic. The digestion of food depends on this acidity.

Human blood has a pH range of 7.36 to 7.44, which is mildly alkaline.

If your blood pH is outside the normal range, your life may be at risk.

This only occurs when the patient has a specific condition, such as diabetes, malnutrition, or alcoholism.

However, diet has no effect on the blood pH.

Maintaining a constant pH level in the blood is vital to one's health.

Your cells will shut down and you will perish rapidly if you do not receive treatment.

Consequently, your body employs a variety of efficient methods to monitor its pH balance. This is the term for acid-base homeostasis.

In fact, the food has a negligible effect on blood pH in healthy individuals, although slight variations may occur within the normal range.

In contrast, sustenance may influence the pH of urine, with varying effects.

Urinary acid excretion is one of the body's primary mechanisms for regulating blood pH.

Your urine will be more acidic immediately after a large meal because your body is eliminating metabolic waste.

Therefore, urine pH is not a reliable indicator of the pH and health of the entire body. Other factors besides your diet may have an impact on your health.

Osteoporosis and substances that produce acid

Osteoporosis is a disorder impacting bone mineral density, as its name suggests.

It is more prevalent in postmenopausal women and can significantly increase your fracture risk.

According to proponents of an alkaline diet, alkaline minerals such as calcium from your bones neutralize acid-forming substances.

Bone mineral density is likely to be lower in those who consume acidic foods, such as the typical Western diet. The acid-ash theory of osteoporosis is frequently mentioned.

However, this theory disregards the significance of your kidneys, which play a crucial role in eliminating acids and sustaining a healthy pH level in the body.

Produced by the kidneys, bicarbonate ions neutralize blood acids and aid in pH regulation.

The pH of the blood is also regulated by the respiratory system. Carbon dioxide and water are expelled from the body when bicarbonate ions bind with blood acids in the kidneys.

The acid-ash hypothesis does not account for the loss of bone protein collagen, which is one of the leading causes of osteoporosis.

Ironically, vitamin C and orthosilicic acid are two acids strongly associated with collagen loss.

Remember that research on the association between dietary acid and bone density or fracture risk is inconsistent. A significant correlation was found despite the fact that numerous observational studies found none.

In more credible clinical studies, it was demonstrated that acid-forming foods have no effect on calcium levels in the body.

As a result of increasing calcium assimilation and activating the IGF-1 hormone, these regimens promote bone and muscle regeneration, thereby improving bone health.

According to these findings, a high-protein, acid-forming diet is likely to enhance bone health rather than damage it.

The Pagen Diet Plan

Combining the best and healthiest aspects of the vegan and paleo diets, the Pegan diet is scientifically proved to aid in weight loss and maintenance. It teaches you how to consume healthily while still enjoying life's small pleasures. This diet will completely alter your perspective and relationship with food, allowing you to effortlessly make healthier decisions for your health and body. If you're just getting started with the plan and have concerns, our Frequently Asked concerns page is here to help. Examine the most frequently inquired Pegan diet plan questions and discover the answers that will help you succeed on the diet.

The Paleo Diet and the Vegan Diet appear to be diametrically opposed. How does this regimen combine the two?

The core to the Pegan diet is what the Paleo Diet and the Vegan Diet have in common, despite their distinctions. Both the Paleo Diet and the Vegan Diet emphasize the importance of eating fresh, natural foods. They also oppose the consumption of refined foods, excessive carbohydrates, and dairy. As long as you adhere to the simple 5-4-3-2-1 method, you will consume the correct foods. It is possible to adhere to both the Paleo and vegan diets.

If I Miss Meals, Will I Lose More Weight?

Although avoiding meals may help you consume fewer calories and lose weight, we do not recommend it for this diet. The 5-4-3-2-1 formula is intended to ensure that you receive all of the essential nutrients on a daily basis; if you neglect meals or portions, your body may not receive all of the sustenance it needs to prosper.

How long do I need to stay on this diet?

This is an all-year nutrition plan. This allows you to lose weight and keep it off permanently, and the best way to achieve this is to adhere to this long-term strategy. Even better if you desire to maintain the regimen for longer than 365 days! With the Pegan diet plan, you will not only receive dietary guidelines, but you will also be taught lifestyle skills, allowing you to continue the diet for as long as you desire.

What beverages are permitted on this diet?

Unless what you're consuming is part of a diet regimen, water is preferable. For instance, one of the breakfast options is a Pegan smoothie consisting of nut butter, almond milk, banana, and vegetables.

Still famished after consuming every portion?

5+ containers of vegetables, 4 carbohydrates, 3 proteins, 2 lipids, and 1 non-dairy product are recommended on Plan 1 of the Pegan Diet. On occasion, however, you could have an active day and still be famished after eating this. The secret is that you are not limited to 5 containers of vegetables; you can consume 5 PLUS! Choose your preferred non-starchy vegetables and consume as many extra servings as you desire! We do not wish for you to be famished.

Is there a calorie limit per day?

Depending on your age, gender, and level of physical activity, the recommended daily number of calories to maintain your weight is typically around 2,000 calories. The good news is that with the Pegan diet plan, calorie counting is unnecessary! You don't have to perform the arduous task of calculating the size of your portions and the number of servings you should consume; this information is provided. Simply recall the 5-4-3-2-1 formula!

I typically do not consume flesh. Do I need to consume flesh to stay on plan?

Although consuming lean meat is a component of the Paleo Diet, you do not need to consume only meat to remain on this diet; legumes, tofu, tempeh, and seeds are acceptable sources of daily protein.

I adore dairy. Should I really quit consuming it?

The Pegan diet does not include dairy on a daily basis. However, it can be difficult to give up dairy forever, so the Pegan diet includes a weekly indulgence day! You desire chocolate dessert on your birthday? Go all out! Craving a slice of mozzarella pizza? Enjoy! You can schedule your indulgence days whenever you'd like and need not stress about giving up your favored foods forever.

Can I consume snacks?

With this regimen, we are only recommending what to consume, not when! You may divide your portions however you see fit, including snacking between meals.

How can I decide what to buy?

We've done all the legwork and compiled a list of items you should seek for at the grocery store.

I'm taking medications. Could this regimen affect their performance?

Certain medications, such as blood thinners and diabetes medications, are affected by the items you eat. Before commencing the diet, if you are taking medications, consult with your doctor to see if a significant change in your diet will affect how your prescriptions work.

After a few days on this regimen, I'm beginning to feel nauseated. What am I to do?

If you begin to notice changes in your health as a result of the diet, you should promptly return to your regular diet and see a doctor. If your symptoms are severe, dial 911 immediately.

HOW THE PEGAN DIET IS CONSTRUED IN CHAPTER 1

The Pegan Grocery List

Now that you know what to expect, here are a few items that should be at the top of your purchasing list:

Your diet should include vegetables with a low glycemic index or carbohydrate content, such as tomatoes, peas, carrots, broccoli, mushrooms, leeks, eggplant, peppers, cauliflower, Brussel sprouts, greens (turnip, mustard, collard, etc.), bamboo stalks, etc.

Look for fruits with a low starch or glycemic index, such as pineapple, mangoes, pears, citrus fruits, dark berries, cherries, apples, oranges, watermelons, etc. Purchase fruits with a high hydration content.

Animal Protein: As long as the flesh is grass-fed and sourced in a sustainable manner, you can consume animal proteins such as whole eggs, poultry, cattle, pork, venison, etc. Additionally, you can consume seafood such as shrimp and halibut.

Healthy Fats: For a Pegan diet, you must consume minimally processed fats from specific sources, such as nuts (except peanuts), seeds (except processed seed oils), unrefined coconut oil, olives, avocados (ensure the avocado and olive oil are cold-pressed), and omega-3 fatty acids (ensure the fish has a low mercury content).

Since you cannot consume dairy products, you are unable to consume conventional butter. There are numerous alternatives to butter, such as vegan butter and pureed avocado. In contrast, some varieties of oils include sesame oil, olive oil, and others. Avoid vegetable oils.

Dairy Replacement: For a Pegan diet, hemp, almond, soy, cashew, hazelnut, and oat are excellent dairy alternatives.

You can include natural carbohydrates such as vanilla, dates, honey, coconut sugar, and maple syrup in your diet.

Except for peanuts, most nuts, such as almonds and hazelnuts, can be ingested. Regarding seeds, chia, pumpkin, and flax seeds provide a nutritious boost.

While legumes are typically discouraged on the Pegan diet, gluten-free, whole legumes are still permitted in limited quantities. The daily allowance should not exceed 75 grams. Pinto legumes, black beans, chickpeas, and lentils are some examples.

Miscellaneous: You may include a variety of miscellaneous ingredients as long as they are natural and low on the glycemic index.

It is advised that you limit your consumption of starchy foods. Even if you consume starches, make sure they come from wholesome sources.

For baked goods, ensure that the ingredients do not contain refined sugar and are gluten-free. Additionally, you can include black rice, quinoa, oats, black beans, and chickpeas.

Supplements: In the case of a Pegan diet, you may take Vitamin D3 and omega-3 fatty acids as supplements. Also available is Vitamin B12.

One-Week Pegan Meal Plan

In addition to vegetables and fruits, a Pegan diet includes seeds, nuts, fish, and sustainably reared proteins. Additionally, you may use gluten-free grains and certain legumes sparingly. Here is a representative itinerary for a week's worth of meals:

Monday

You can prepare a vegetable omelet with a simple green salad topped with olive oil for breakfast.

You may choose a basic salad with avocado, strawberries, and legumes for lunch.

Monday Tuesday Wednesday Thursday Friday Saturday

Dinner options include wild salmon fillets with lemon vinaigrette, steamed asparagus, and roasted carrots.

Breakfast: sweet potato crostini garnished with pumpkin seeds, avocado slices, and lemon vinaigrette.

Prepare a Bento box containing blackberries, fermented pickles, fresh vegetable spears, cut poultry, and hard-boiled eggs for lunch.

Evening meal: black beans, tomato, bell pepper, scallions, and almonds stir-fried with bell peppers.

Breakfast should consist of a green smoothie containing hemp seeds, almond butter, kale, and apple.

Vegetable stir-fry leftovers from Tuesday make for a simple supper. Dinner consists of vegetable kebabs, prawns grilled on skewers, and black rice pilaf.

This morning's ideal breakfast would consist of chia seed and coconut pudding with fresh blueberries and hazelnuts.

The best option for a simple meal on this day is a mixed green salad with cider vinaigrette, grilled chicken, cucumber, and avocado. Dinner: Roasted beet salad with sliced hazelnuts, Brussels sprouts, and pumpkin seeds.

Breakfast consists of braised vegetables, kimchi, and eggs sautéed in butter.

Lunch will consist of vegetable stew and lentils with a side of cantaloupe slices.

Friday's dinner will consist of a salad containing grass-fed beef fillets, guacamole, jicama, and radishes.

Sunday

Breakfast on the weekends should consist of overnight cereals, berries, hazelnuts, chia seeds, and cashew milk.

For supper, consume the vegetable stew and lentils from yesterday. Saturday night's supper should consist of pork loin roasted with quinoa, herbs, and stewed vegetables.

Breakfast on a Sunday should consist of a straightforward vegetable omelet and green salad.

Enjoy the Thai-style salad rolls with citrus slices and cashew cream dressing for lunch.

Dinner: pork loin and vegetables from the previous night's dinner.

Benefits Of The Vegan Diet To Health

Numerous individuals who have followed the Pegan diet have reported a variety of additional medical benefits in addition to weight loss or weight management. Some of these additional medical benefits include:

Reduced risk of heart disease

The most notable benefit of a nutritious diet is a robust heart. People who consume a diet rich in newly grown foods, whole cereals, vegetables, nuts, seeds, and lean proteins appear to have a significantly reduced risk of developing heart-related conditions such as heart failure, stroke, and hypertension.

Reduces blood glucose levels

Numerous investigations have demonstrated that a sound, adjusted, and healthy eating routine can help people with diabetes and elevated glucose levels prevent, manage, and in some cases cure diabetes, including type 2 diabetes, without the need for daily medications.

Reduced Risk for Alzheimer's

Due to the high number of cell-reinforcing properties, a healthful diet rich in newly grown crops from the ground has been demonstrated repeatedly. Reduces a person's risk of developing Alzheimer's disease and other psychological diseases and conditions.

Weight Management

Restricting poor food types (processed, sugary, or food sources rich in rancid fats) has demonstrated benefits to a person's waistline, with numerous studies demonstrating that those who eat a healthy, balanced, and nutritious diet can lose excess fat rather than muscle more rapidly and sustain this weight loss for longer durations than those who don't.

Pegan Cheat Sheet (CHAPTER 5)

A basic guide to what you should consume.

Eat Much

Non-dull vegetables

Low-glycemic fruits and vegetables (berries, kiwis, citrus, etc.)

Eggs

Low mercury fish (such as salmon, mackerel, sardines, and anchovies).

Consume a Moderate Amount

Low-glycemic cereals, such as brown rice or quinoa (up to a half-cup per meal).

Vegetables and beans (up to 1 cup per day)

Natural, grass-fed meat and poultry (up to four to six ounces per entrée)

Healthy lipids (olive oil, avocado oil, copra oil, ghee, margarine)

Consume slightly bland vegetables

High-glycemic fruits and vegetables (grapes, melons, cherries, etc.)

Seeds and nuts

Goat or sheep's milk dairy products

Infrequent Treats

Dried plant preparations

Juices

Sugar Liquor (no more than two to five servings per week).

Abstain from Handled dietary sources

Cow's milk dairy, excluding margarine and ghee.

Oils derived from plants (canola, maize, soybean, sunflower, etc.).

Sources of Consumable Food on the Pegan Diet

The essential nutritional category for the Pegan diet is vegetables and organic products, which must account for 75% of your total daily consumption.

Low-glycemic plant foods, such as berries and brightly colored vegetables, must be highlighted to limit your glucose response. Individuals who have successfully achieved solid glycemic control prior to beginning a diet may consume limited quantities of mild vegetables and saccharine natural products. People adhering to the Pegan diet are encouraged to consume banquets that prioritize whole food sources, or food sources that have remained true to their structure with minimal processing prior to being transported to a kitchen.

Rye Sourdough Bread

INGREDIENTS

- 100 g natural sourdough

- 1 tbsp. salt

- 1200 ml water

- 1500 g whole grain rye flour and flour to work with

1. In a mixing bowl, combine 400 g flour, 600 ml lukewarm water, and the sourdough.

2. Cover and set aside for 4 hours in a warm spot.

3. Then, with the remaining flour and salt, knead all together thoroughly.

4. Knead for 10 minutes or until the dough is firm and malleable, adding flour as required.

5. Cover with a bowl and set aside to rest for 1 hour.

6. Then, on a floured work surface, knead the dough thoroughly and form it into a loaf.

7. Place in a proofing basket after thoroughly flouring. Allow for another 30 minutes of resting time after covering.

8. In the oven, place a refractory bowl filled with water.

9. Turn the bread carefully out of the basket and onto a baking sheet lined with parchment paper.

10.   In a preheated oven, bake in the lower third for 30-40 minutes.

11.   Let the loaf to cool, slice and serve.

Crafted Crunchy Muesli

INGREDIENT

- 15 chopped walnuts

- 2 tbsp sesame seeds

- 2 tbsp sunflower seeds

Raisins

- 2/3 lb (300g) mixed flakes (oats, spelt, wheat and rye)
- 4 tablespoons liquid honey (if your honey is a bit solid, you'll have to heat it a few minutes to soften)

- 1 tbsp vegetable oil

INSTRUCTIONS

1. The oven should be preheated to 360° Fahrenheit and the baking sheet should be oiled before beginning.
2. In a large skillet, heat the cereal flakes and almonds. Dry roast them for 5-7 minutes over medium heat. Avoid burning by stirring regularly. When you smell the toasted flakes, you know it's done.
3. Cool the flakes in a plate. In a mixing dish, combine liquid honey, oil, & salt A medium speed electric mixer
4. works nicely.
5. On a baking sheet, distribute the ingredients evenly.
6. Preheat the oven to 360°F (180°) and bake for 20 minutes.
7. Allow to cool before breaking into pieces for your crunchy muesli. Add

the raisins and store in an airtight container.

Salad Of Refreshing Watermelon

- 3 tablespoons lime juice
- 1 cup sliced red onion, cut lengthwise
- 15 cups cubed watermelon
- 3 cups cubed English cucumber
- 1 (8 ounces) package feta cheese, crumbled
- ½ cup chopped fresh cilantro
- cracked black pepper
- sea salt

Directions

1. Pour lime juice over red onions in a small dish.
2. Allow marinating while putting the salad together.
3. In a large mixing basin, gently incorporate the watermelon,

cucumber, feta cheese, and cilantro. Black pepper to taste.
4. Just before serving, toss the watermelon salad with the marinated onions and season with salt.

Overnight Fruit Chia Oatmeal

Ingredients:

Maple syrup, or a different sweetener, to taste

1 cup frozen berries of choice or smoothie leftovers

Toppings:

Yogurt

Berries

1/2 cup Quaker Oats rolled oats

1/4 cup chia seeds

1 cup milk or water

Pinch of salt and cinnamon

1. Combine the oats, seeds, milk, salt, and cinnamon in a container with a cover and chill overnight.

2. Blend the berries in a blender on the day of serving.

3. Toss the oats with the berry puree, then top with yogurt and additional berries, nuts, honey, or any other garnish you like. Enjoy!

Green Morning Smoothie

- 1 orange, peeled, and cut into segments

- 1 cup unsweetened nondairy milk

- 1 cup ice

- 1/2 Banana, sliced

- 2 cups spinach

- 1 cup sliced berries of your choosing, fresh or frozen

1. In a blender, combine all the ingredients.

2. Starting with the blender at low speed, begin blending the smoothie, gradually increasing blender speed until smooth.

3. Serve immediately.

152

Toast Topped With Avocado, Egg, And Sprouts.

Ingredients:

- 1 egg
- 1/4 cup sprouts
- 1 slice bread
- 1/2 avocado
- **salt and pepper to taste**

Preparation:

1. Toast the bread until it is crispy and golden brown.
2. Meanwhile, bring a small pot of water to a boil.

3. Carefully add the egg and easy cook for about 10 minutes for a medium-boiled egg.

4. Remove the egg from the pot and peel away the shell.

5. Spread the avocado onto the toast.

6. Slice the egg and place the slices on top of the avocado.

7. Top with sprouts and season with salt and pepper to taste.

Easy Baked Avocado Eggs

- 4 large eggs

- ¼ teaspoon freshly ground black pepper

- 2 medium or large avocados, halved and pitted

1. Preheat the oven to 450°F.

2. Scoop out some of the pulp from the avocado halves, leaving enough space to fit an egg, reserving the pulp for Easy Guacamole

3. Line an 8-by-8-inch baking pan with foil. Place the avocado halves in the pan to fit snugly in a single layer, folding the foil around the outer avocados to prevent tipping.

4. Crack 1 egg into each avocado half; season with pepper. Bake, uncovered, until the whites are set and the egg yolks

are cooked to your desired doneness, 12 to 15 minutes.

5. Remove from the oven and let rest for 5 minutes before serving.